The Auto Immune Solution

Learn how to Prevent and Overcome Inflammatory Diseases and Live a Pain-Free Life

Table of Contents

trademark owner. All trademarks and brands within this book are for clarifying purposes only and are the owned by the owners themselves, not affiliated with this document.

Introduction

I want to thank you and congratulate you for downloading the book, *"The Auto Immune Solution."*

This book contains proven steps and strategies on how to repair your digestive system and alleviate any autoimmune illnesses.

Read on to find out what exactly happens in your own immune system. Learn how the food you eat will affect your entire body, and not just your stomach. As we take you through this guide you will soon have an understanding of:

- How the food you eat can cause autoimmune diseases such as arthritis, asthma, and many other conditions.

- Learn how the condition of a leaky gut can, and will lead to other parts of your body becoming inflamed, and not functioning correctly.

- Understand how you can start to repair a leaky gut, and find out what you can do to reverse this effect?

- Yes, it is possible to heal yourself!

We will discuss Functional Medicine and the Myer's 4R Program, as one way to help your leaky gut heal.

In this book you will learn which foods will not only reverse leaky gut, but will also prevent it.

Finally, we will discuss alternative medicine for additional treatment of inflammation diseases, and then finish with an in depth look at a gluten free diet.

Thanks again for downloading this book, I hope you enjoy it!

Chapter 1 What is the Immune System?

Defense Mechanisms

Considering that we are surrounded by billions of bacteria bugs and viruses, it is no wonder that the human body has a complex system for fighting them off and keeping your body, for the most part, safe from harm. This complex system is known as the immune system

The human defense mechanisms are extremely complicated, and very complex, starting with the skin as the first line of defense. The skin does more than simply cover your body frame. Your skin is only one small part of your autoimmune system, which is an amazing and natural mechanism that, for the most part, helps to keep us fit and healthy and safe from harm. Sometimes, things can go wrong, and when that happens it can seriously damage your health.

Blood is also on the frontline of your defenses. It contains certain types of white blood cells that fight against pathogens, or toxins, that can get into your bloodstream. Most common of these are Phagocytes and lymphocytes. These are the "Generals," in the immune system, and direct the body's response to infectious micro-organisms, and other damaging foreign bodies.

Another important element of the immune system is your lymphatic nodes, also known as lymphatic glands. These are small glands around the human body that are connected by a network of lymph channels. You have around 600 of these, which form in little clusters at certain points throughout the body, such as the arm pits, the groin and the neck. This is known as the lymphatic system. These also contain the lymphocytes and antibodies that help the body fight infectious diseases.

We can further divide the immune system into two parts, one that you are born with, and one that you develop as you mature.

Innate Immunity

Your innate immunity, also known as non-specific immunity, is your first line of defense. It is a physical and chemical deterrent to harmful pathogens that may attempt to infiltrate your system. The skin is your outer barrier, not only does it provide you with a waterproof covering, it also helps prevent invasion of microscopic organisms from attacking your inner body. Where there are breaks in the skin, such as the mouth and nose, they usually have a defensive wall to help stop bacterial entities from entering the body. In the case of the nose, it is a mucus membrane and nasal hair, and in the mouth your saliva can kill off many bacteria that enter that way. Those that survive are often killed off by the gastric juices in your stomach. Inflammation is another innate immunity mechanism of your body, fighting off invading antigens and helping heal damaged tissue.

Specific Immunity

This system is understood to be a developed system, unlike the innate immune system, which has defenses present at birth, the specific immune system needs to develop a response to invading pathogens. This is your "targeted" response to those pathogens that manage to get past your innate immunity. This is where the white blood cells, and your lymph gland system work well together. Once any pathogens or toxins enter your body, it triggers your immune system to respond. How it responds is dependent on the type of white blood cells called upon. In the case of Phagocytes, they ingest the invading organism, but if it is the lymphocytes, then they create antibodies to kill the invaders. It is this procedure as to why we sometimes do not suffer certain infections repeatedly. Even though previous antibodies may be in our system again, our t-cells have already developed a response to them. Meaning they can deal with them quickly, often with reduced symptoms, and sometimes without any symptoms at all. You have built up a specific immunity as your body matures.

Lymphatic System

The lymphatic system has a number of important functions, the main one being draining fluid from your body and filtering bacteria from the bloodstream. The lymphatic system consists of lymph vessels, such as the tonsils, spleen and thymus.

The thymus is a crucial element in the building of your immune system. It is a gland that is situated in the front part of your chest, and it is only active in the years up to puberty. Once into adulthood, it starts to shrink until it is eventually replaced by fatty tissue. Its function is to develop and train T-lymphocytes, also known as t-cells. It is these t-cells that will learn to defend your body form invading pathogens, such as viruses and bacteria, as you mature. Part of this training is to teach the t-cells to know the difference between invading antigens, and the body's own antigens. This is a testing for the autoimmunity system to ensure that those which attach to the body's own antigens. are rejected.

The spleen is the largest of the lymphatic organs, in your body. This is situated near the ribs, on the left and is about the size of an adult clenched fist. Its main functions are the purifying of blood, and storing of white blood cells. The spleen consists of two different types of tissue; red and white pulp, with each having its own unique function. The white pulp is lymphatic tissue and mainly made up of white blood cells, who's role it is to produce and grow t-lymphocytes that are then used in fighting pathogens. The red pulp is a network of blood filled channels which filter out the harmful pathogens from the blood, as well as removing damaged and old blood cells. This is where your storage of platelets will develop, that will help your blood to clot. These platelets will be released at times of extreme bleeding.

Chapter 2 Autoimmune Disorder

Sometimes, your body can get it wrong, become confused, and the very white blood cells that are there to protect you and destroy harmful antigens, can turn on the body's own healthy tissue. When this happens, it is known as Autoimmune Disease. This condition affects many people from different walks of life, but women are more susceptible, especially those who have had children, with 75% of autoimmune cases in the U.S, being female. No one is certain why this happens, though many scientists believe that certain drugs and viruses bring it about, especially with those that have the gene that predisposes them to the disorder. Although in recent studies, some scientists believe that diet is a major factor in developing autoimmune disease, and this **study** shows that there is a link with consuming junk food. They conclude that a diet enriched with refined salt, is a contributor to autoimmune disease.

Autoimmune disorder can result in serious health problems, such as:

- Destruction of healthy tissue.

- Abnormal growths.

- Altering organ function.

There are over 80 autoimmune diseases, some are quite rare, whereas others are more common, such as:

- Rheumatoid Arthritis.

- Psoriasis.

- Type 1 Diabetes.

- Celiac Disease.

- Irritable Bowel Disease (I.B.S).

- Hay Fever.

- Multiple Sclerosis.

There are two categories of autoimmune disease: localized or organ specific, and systematic, where multiple areas in the body can be affected.

Although localized autoimmune disease is specific to one organ, a patient may often suffer from autoimmune disease in other specific organs at the same time. Further, whilst organ specific may be restricted to certain organs, often the effects of the disease may also appear in other parts in the body. For example Diabetes type 1 patients may suffer with problems in their eyes, kidneys, and muscles, as well as many other complications.

Typical symptoms for someone suffering from autoimmune disease is prolonged inflammation, causing pain, heat and swelling.

Chapter 3 What is Inflammation?

Inflammation is actually a function of your body attempting to protect you, and is a part of the innate immune system. It is a generic reaction of your immune system, to fight off harmful bacteria that have damaged tissue. When this happens, those damaged cells release chemicals that cause blood to leak into the surrounding area, isolating the foreign substance from causing further damage to other tissue. These chemicals further attract the white blood cell variation, Phagocytes, which will then digest the damaged tissue and the invading pathogen. Therefore, inflammation is an important part of your immune system, and helps to stop infections from spreading to other areas in your body. Inflammation is essential for repairing damaged tissue, and without it, the damaged areas would never heal and would eventually decay.

Classical signs of inflammation to the body are:

- Swelling.

- Redness.

- Pain.

- Hot skin.

- Numbness.

Your body does try to balance the amount of inflammation. If there is too little inflammation, then then the invading pathogen may cause widespread tissue damage, equally if there is too much inflammation, then this can result in a number of serious diseases, such as peritonitis, rheumatoid arthritis, hay fever and in some extreme cases, cancer.

Inflammation is categorized as either:

ACUTE - When the body naturally retaliates against harmful bacteria, your immune system will trigger into action. It will create an improved blood flow to the infected or damaged area with an increase of white blood cells to kill the invading pathogen and repair the damaged tissue. Acute inflammation lasts only for a few days.

CHRONIC - Sometimes the inflammation can go on for longer, which may be due to the immune system not eradicating the infectious antibodies. Chronic inflammation can go on to cause other diseases in the body, such as arthritis and osteoporosis.

Inflammation is not an infection, though it may have been brought about to fight off an infection in the first place. The chronic stages of inflammation mean that your body is now fighting its own cells, thinking they are invaders. When this happens, it is classed as a type of autoimmune disease.

Studies have shown that 25 percent of autoimmunity patients have the symptoms through genetic causation. However, 75 percent have contracted these effects through environmental factors, such as leaky gut, diet, toxins and stress. With over 80 different autoimmune diseases, there can be periods of painful symptoms and then other times of little or no symptoms at all. These are known as "remission," and "flare ups." The reasons as to why this happens, is not really understood, but there are triggers that can cause "flare ups," such as bacteria or viruses, medication, chemicals and other non-specific causes.

Different parts of the body can be affected and often more than one:

- Joints.

- Muscles.

- Skin.

- Blood cells and vessels.

- Tissue.

- Glands.

Equally, it can be argued that different factors can contribute to the condition leading up to an autoimmunity breakdown:

- Diet, such as grains and gluten.

- How the gut reacts to our diet, leading to conditions such as leaky gut.

- Toxins in food and the environment.

- Stress and hormones.

- Infections, bacteria and viruses.

Chapter 4 What is Leaky Gut?

The gut is home to literally trillions of micro-organisms, and over 400 diverse and different forms of bacteria reside in the gut. These micro-organisms and bacteria, contribute to more than simply digesting your food. They are a major contributor to your immune system, helping you fight infections as well as regulating your metabolism. Deficiencies in this gut flora are linked to many diseases, including some autoimmune diseases, such as Inflammatory Bowel Disease (IBS), and diabetes type 1. There has even been evidence, shown in this study, that autistic children have a high level of gastrointestinal problems, that can be produced by poorly regulated bacteria in the gut.

Recently, several alternative nutritional experts believe that many of the autoimmune diseases are caused by problems in the gut, especially with an abnormal amount of gut bacteria present. It is from this where the term "leaky gut", also known as increased intestinal permeability, comes from. The wall of the gut, or intestine, is meant as a barrier to stop particles of food from leaking into our circulatory system, but sometimes a build-up of toxins from a poor diet, or medication, can cause damage to this lining and reduce its effectiveness. When this happens, foreign invaders enter our system, which in turn causes an immune reaction as the body responds to this condition. This can result in severe health conditions. Indeed, they argue that leaky gut syndrome has been linked, scientifically, as an influence of diseases that you would not normally associate with gut problems. The gut lining should act as a barrier to keep out digestive toxins from the rest of your body, but it has been weakened by bacteria, resulting in particles of food actually managing to pass through and enter the bloodstream.

Common Symptoms for those who suffer leaky gut syndrome include:

- Digestive problems such as excessive wind, diarrhea, Irritable Bowel Syndrome (IBS).

- Seasonal allergies, such as hay fever.

- Chronic fatigue and poor memory.

- Mood swings and depression.

- Food allergies.

- Candida infection (Thrush).

So, what is the solution to leaky gut syndrome?

Initially, it is necessary to repair the damaged lining to the stomach. To do this, you must abstain from certain foods and any medication that has been identified as an instigator to this problem.

Here are some of the recommendations for repairing the damage to your gut wall.

- A 14 day detox period is ideal, eliminating the usual suspects that have been identified as a cause to leaky gut syndrome, such as gluten, dairy, sugar and alcohol.

- Wherever possible, AVOID the following medication: antibiotics, anti-inflammatories and anti-acid tablets. All of these will kill much of the good bacteria in your gut lining, and allow the bad bacteria to increase and attack the lining of the wall, in effect rotting it.

- LIMIT your intake of sugars, processed foods, saturated and trans fats and animal protein. They all carry the bad bacteria, which again, will overcome the good bacteria in your stomach.

- INCREASE fiber rich foods in your daily diet, they are an excellent source of nutrition and have many health benefits, such as reducing cholesterol, lowering blood sugars and helping with constipation. Such foods are:

- Vegetables and fruits (in particular fermented vegetables such as pickles).

- Coconut products, including the flesh, milk and oil.

- Sprouted seeds, such as chia, flax and hemp.

- Raw garlic and onions are rich in natural antioxidants, which can prevent some cells from becoming infected, by blocking out certain chemical reactions known as "free radicals," which are damaged cells.

- Certain herbs, such as licorice root (see chapter 6 on herbs).

- Don't forget to increase your fluid intake to account for the more fibrous diet, but ensure that these are no-sugar liquids. This will help to keep the fiber moving healthily along your digestive system. The more fiber you eat, then the more liquid you should drink, this can be in the form of teas, particularly herbal teas, milk, decaffeinated coffee and non-sugar fruit juices.

- DIGEST probiotics daily, such as yogurt, dark chocolate, green pickles, sauerkraut and any other foods that are rich in probiotics. The bacteria in these foods will help to reduce inflammation caused by leaky gut as they invade the bad types of bacteria present in the gut.

There are tests that you can ask your doctor about, to measure the level of bacteria in your gut. This might give you an idea of what is going on in your own digestive system.

Chapter 5 Treatment: Functional Medicine

There is a general acceptance among professionals, that there is no cure for autoimmune disease, only treatments that can help to control the flare up symptoms. Sometimes though, these treatments can cause more problems than they can solve. Here are some suggestions of possible scenarios of what a doctor trying to treat autoimmune conditions, may prescribe for you:

- Pain medication - certain types of pain medication can have a negative effect on the stomach, by killing the good bacteria, especially when taken without food.

- There is also the option of anti-inflammatory medication, which is often prescribed for inflammation, swelling and pain in joints, as in arthritis. Again, certain anti-inflammatory medications can actually cause problems in the stomach which may lead to the lining of the stomach bleeding.

- Meanwhile, they may encourage you to also try vitamin supplements, or hormone replacement therapies (for certain conditions only). All unbalancing your body's natural immune system.

Still not working?

- So, they may suggest trying immunosuppressive medication, which involves actually suppressing your immunity system.

  Still suffering?

- Then they may suggest that you could always consider a blood transfusion (for certain conditions only).

At the end of the day, despite some of these very intensive treatments, there will be no guarantee that you will be symptom free, or cured.

So, what is the autoimmune solution about?

First, you need to learn the root causes. Once you understand that, you might be able to prevent this from happening to your body, or if you already suffer inflammation in some form, then perhaps you can heal yourself. Only once you have discovered the causes of your problems, can you learn how to start reversing the effects of such life restricting, and painful conditions.

It is hard for anyone in pain, not to reach for the help of conventional medicines, such as pain killers in the form of drugs. Yet, there are other ways to start reversing the effects of your immune system, once it is attacking itself. Ask yourself, what has caused it to do this in the first place? It is becoming a popular understanding, amongst alternative medicine practitioners and some traditional doctors, that the gut is the "first port of call." This is where your nutrition input first arrives, and this is where it starts to be broken down, or enters the bloodstream. It makes sense to ensure that all is working well in your digestive system, because if it is not functioning correctly, then leaky gut syndrome could be the cause of the breakdown in your autoimmune system.

If you suffer from any of the following conditions, then you need to read on:

- Seasonal allergies, such as Hay fever.

- Uncontrolled weight gain.

- Hormonal imbalance, leading to lethargy and mood swings.

- Inflammation, such as arthritis.

- Digestive problems from gas to Irritable Bowl Syndrome (IBS)

- Osteoporosis in women, (particularly at menopausal stages when hormones are imbalanced in your body).

15

Some scientists believe that if the gut is healthy, then the rest of the body will start to heal, because the gut is the mainstay of your health condition. They further believe that if the gastrointestinal (GI) tract is problematic, then problems elsewhere in the body are inevitable. A healthy gut is a healthy person, it was Hippocrates over 2000 years ago who believed that all diseases start in the gut. Perhaps we should have heeded those words sooner.

Chapter 6 Treatment: Alternative Therapies

You don't have to rely on traditional medicinal treatments in the form of an array of drugs, to help cure your autoimmune disease. There are alternative solutions that can be considered, as well as the dietary intake we have suggested. Please note, you should not stop taking any medication prescribed for you by a medical practitioner, without first seeking proper advice.

One such alternative approach to helping with auto-immune disease, and also including leaky gut, is known as "The Myers Guide," and it starts with "The 4 R Program:"

REMOVE - all toxic foods from your diet, such as sugar, caffeine, dairy and processed products that can be high in sugars and salts. Any foods that are known to disrupt the digestive process.

REPLACE - adding back restorative ingredients to the dietary intake, by eating more protein and healthy fats, all of which will function in the gut without causing any damage and will encourage the good bacteria in your gut flora.

REINOCULATE - adding probiotics to the gut, which will encourage healthy bacteria growth, needed to fight the bad bacteria, which we know causes gut leak in the first place.

REPAIR - adding amino acids, zinc, omega oils and certain herbs and vitamins, such as aloe vera, that will repair any damage already done to the gut lining and speed up its recovery.

By following this 4 part guide, you will be well on your way to repairing your leaky gut, which many alternative practitioners believe is a major cause of auto-immune disease.

HERBS

Herbs have long been recognized as a good source of healing, and have been used for millennia. They are tried, tested and used in many cultures such as Chinese, Indian and African. There are various herbs that will help you in the healing process of the damaged tissue from leaky gut:

- Milk thistle and dandelion root contain flavonoids and help to detoxify the liver, which may be overloaded with toxins.

- Slippery elm helps coat the stomach lining.

- Licorice root helps balance cortisol levels.

- Echinacea provides a welcoming boost to your immune system.

- Peppermint and chamomile tea sooth the symptoms of leaky gut. Peppermint assists in ridding the gut of those overwhelming bad bacteria that are causing so much trouble in your intestines. You can also take peppermint in capsule form, as it is filled with peppermint oil. Chamomile has a more soothing effect and will help to relieve any cramps, bloating or wind, which in turn will alleviate stress as you start to feel better.

- Ginger helps to soothe inflammation in the stomach

- Turmeric is a powerful anti-inflammatory spice

- Garlic lowers yeast overgrowth, helping with your cholesterol levels, as well as blood pressure.

All of these can easily be added to your cooking, not only increasing your dishes' health benefit, but also improving its flavor.

CHIROPRACTIC TREATMENT

Many people choose chiropractic care for the treatment of autoimmune disease. Chiro-practitioners are well established, and it is one of the largest alternative medical professions. They believe that many diseases originate from the nervous system, and much of their treatment is in the area of the spine. They will manipulate this area by applying force to muscles, bones and joints. This, they argue, all helps to alleviate the symptoms of inflammation in various areas of your body. Whilst it may cause some minor discomfort initially it is not a painful treatment. Chiropractors may also massage soft tissue and provide you with a rehabilitation program that you will integrate into your lifestyle. This may involve advice on diet and exercise, all aimed at improving your health.

ACUPUNCTURE

Acupuncture is an ancient form of alternative medicine and a major element of Chinese medicine. It is also practiced in other Eastern Asian cultures, such as Japan and India. Acupuncture involves the stimulation of certain points in the body, with very fine needles. These are inserted into the body at certain crucial points, and is backed up with scientific evidence as being successful for certain conditions. How acupuncture works is dependent upon your culture. From a western perspective, the needles stimulate nerves to produce endorphins, which are the body's natural form of pain relievers. Those from eastern cultures, where it is more widely practiced, believe it is a more spiritual experience, and related to Qi, the source of all energy, and in humans this is related to their health and wellbeing. In all cultures it is used for many conditions including inflammatory ones, such as osteoarthritis, back pains, headaches and asthma.

HYPNOSIS

Contrary to popular belief, this is not a sleep induced state, but more of a trance, a mental state of the mind. The subject is still aware and alert, almost likened to meditation. In reality we all of us do our own version of hypnosis every day of our lives. We may watch a movie or read a book, and totally cut out what is happening around us. Done correctly, the subject is open to suggestions, as there is an element of access to the subconscious mind. Remember, that this part of the brain is an amazing organ; we breath, walk and talk subconsciously. This is the real part of the brain that manipulates your body to function, without you even having to think about it. Scientists believe that in hypnosis, this part of the brain is alert, and it is a part of the brain that we cannot delve into if we are in our normal state of mind. It is by manipulating the subconscious, that therapists are able to assist with problems in life, such as habits, fears, pain. Masters of meditation can do this by themselves, and it is believed they are able to heal themselves by entering a deep meditative state.

These are some of the more common alternative treatments for helping with symptoms of autoimmune disease. Some are supported by scientific trials, others have less authority. For many sufferers of inflammatory pain, all these methods can help to reduce the symptoms. Sometimes the best method is to use conventional medicine, as prescribed by your doctor, especially IF it has no adverse side effects, and you could use complimentary treatments in conjunction. That way you get the best of both worlds.

Chapter 7 Gluten Free Diet

Increasingly it is being considered that gluten in the diet may be a cause of some of the symptoms of autoimmune disease. There is growing evidence that gluten is a major contributor to autoimmune thyroid disease (AITD). AITD is the condition where the immune system believes that the thyroid glands are a threat to the body, so go on to create antibodies to attack it. This is very similar to autoimmune disease. There are many studies showing a clear link, in fact the evidence is so great, that all patients displaying signs of AITD are regularly screened for gluten intolerance. Because of the similarities between the two diseases, many have linked gluten intolerance as an actual cause of autoimmune disease.

What is it in gluten that causes so many problems?

All gluten, including that found in grains and flours damage our intestinal lining, therefore increasing the risk of leaky gut and inhibit nutritional absorption. Increasing evidence indicates that for some people gluten can trigger an autoimmune response that actually causes damage the body.

The fundamental foods that contain gluten are:

- Wheat.

- Grains such as Barley, Malt and Rye.

- Oats can become contaminated, so avoid unless labeled "Gluton Free,"

These basic ingredients can be found in an array of processed foods that should be avoided, such as:

- Bread

- Beer

- Cakes

- Cereals

- Candy

- Sauces

- Snack foods

- Soups

Look for the "Gluten Free," label when purchasing these types of foods.

Also be aware that products marked "Wheat Free," does not necessarily mean "Gluten Free," as gluten is also present in other foods (see fundamental foods above).

Foods made from certain grains are safe to eat in small amounts, such as:

- Rice

- Corn

However, a gluten free diet can leave you with certain deficiencies leading to low levels of certain key nutrients, such as iron, calcium, fiber and more, so you will need to counter balance this in other foods, or you may need to take these as supplements, but always seek medical advice first.

Conditions that may benefit from a gluten free diet:

- Autism.

- Celiac disease.

- Those with Wheat or Gluten allergies.

- Multiple Sclerosis.

- Thyroid disease.

- Attention Deficit Hyperactivity Disorder (ADHD).

- Osteoporosis.

Most of these conditions have been shown to be alleviated when switching to a gluten free diet.

There are other conditions whereby a gluten free diet has also helped to alleviate symptoms:

- Skin problems such as rashes, dermatitis, eczema.

- Fatigue.

- Digestive problems, such as IBS, gas, constipation and diarrhea.

- Headaches, such as migraine.

- Joint and muscle pains.

- Mood swings and depression.

- Tingling of hands and feet.

- Weight gain and weight loss, that cannot seem to be controlled.

Foods that are safe to eat, and don't contain gluten, include:-

- Fruit and vegetables.

- Almond flour.

- Millet.

- Potatoes.

- Soy flour.

Starting a gluten free lifestyle is not going to be easy, especially for those who enjoy products high in gluten, such as bread, cereals, pasta, candy and many fast foods. The evidence is beginning to mount, that gluten may not be entirely good for us, and some argue that we could all benefit by limiting, if not completely removing it from our diet.

Conclusion

This book is a guide to helping you heal yourself by understanding what is happening in your own body. Understanding the mechanism of your digestive system will give you a spring board to alleviating autoimmune symptoms, such as inflammation, from the rest of your body.

You can start slowly. It does not have to be done in a day. But, start you must, to introduce some changes into your diet so you can go on to live a healthier lifestyle, free of pain.

Lastly, if you enjoyed reading this book, I would greatly appreciate your book review on Amzon.com

Good luck.

Preview Of '*Juicing for Health: The Essential Guide To Healing Common Diseases with Proven Juicing Recipes and Staying Healthy For Life*' by Donna Cavanaugh

Acne

Lemon Twist (morning drink)

Ingredients

- 1 Lemon
- 1 cup hot water

Carrot Clear

Ingredients

- 8 Carrots
- 2 stalks Celery
- ½ cup Watercress

Dandelion Leaves Juice

Ingredients

- 1 handful Dandelion leaves
- 1 Apple

- 1 Red Beet
- 1 Lemon

Explanation

Acne is an inflammatory disease of the sebaceous glands and hair follicles of the skin that is marked by the eruption of pimples or pustules, especially on the face. Fresh lemon, dandelion, carrots, celery, beets and apples purify the blood, removing metabolic waste and changing pH from acidic to alkaline

Allergies

Red Velvet

Ingredients

- 4 Carrots
- 2 stalks Celery
- 1 cup Pineapple
- 1 thumb Ginger
- ½ Red Beet

Green Beast

Ingredients

- 2 Apples
- 3 stalks Celery
- 1 Cucumber
- 1 thumb Ginger
- ½ Lemon (with rind)
- 1 Lime (with rind)
- 1 bunch Parsley
- 2 cups Spinach

Explanation

Allergies are triggered where the responses to allergens that your body absorbs from the environment or from your diet, causing heightened immune system responses, usually with inappropriate levels of inflammation or irritation. Pineapple contains the enzyme bromelain, which is widely used by German physicians to treat inflammation and swelling of the nose, ear, and sinuses. Recent scientific research has proven that ginger can be used for therapies of various illnesses due to its antioxidant effects, its ability to inhibit the formation of inflammatory compounds, and its anti-inflammatory effects.

Anemia

Beet Anemia

Ingredients

- 4 Carrots
- 2 stalks Celery
- 2 Red Beets
- 1 handful Blackberries
- 2 oz Lettuce

Explanation

Anemia is a condition where the number of red blood cells or concentrations of hemoglobin are low. Iron is the foundation for hemoglobin, the molecule which is responsible for the transport of oxygen. In Europe, beet juice has been used for centuries as a treatment for anemia, due to its high content of iron, folic acid, Vitamin B1, B2, B6, and vitamins A & C.

To read more, please visit Amazon.com

Other Book Recommendations:

Clean Gut: The Breakthrough Plan for Eliminating the Root Cause of Disease and Revolutionizing Your Health by Alejandro Junger

GMO Free Diet: The Ultimate Guide on Avoiding GMO Foods and keeping Your Family Healthy with a GMO Free Diet by Michael Skinner